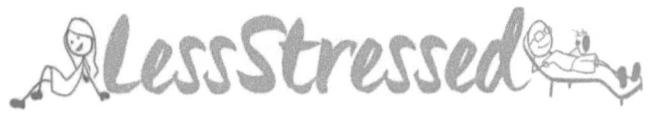

How to be LessStressed™

From Survive and Strive to Revive and Thrive

by

I0436753

Dr Julie Leoni

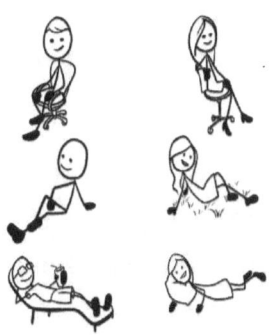

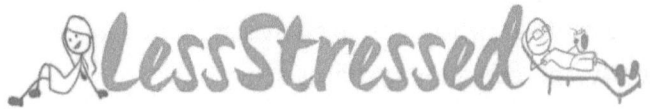

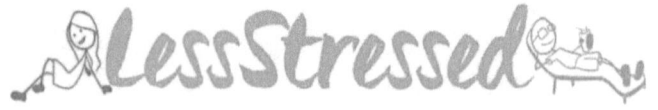

Introduction

This is an book about how to be less stressed. I can't promise that you will never feel stressed again, but if you practice using the tools in this book, then when stress comes knocking, you will know how to send it packing.

How do I know? Because these are the tools and processes I use every day one to one with clients and on the various training courses I run for schools and organisations. I know these tools work because people tell me they do. Also I have seen people change; they look and behave so differently once the stress has gone.

Often when I meet clients they are tearful, agitated or angry. Sometimes everyone is to blame but themselves and often they can see no way out, which of course increases their stress. When you are stressed you feel overwhelmed by the slightest thing and making decisions that could help you seems impossible as when you are stressed you can't think clearly and everything seems scary.

I have coached and trained young people to manage exam pressures, partners who are flailing in the face of relationships issues and employees overwhelmed by work. These tools work.

Working with stress provides you with an opportunity to make real, healthy and inspired changes to your life. As you read this book and try out the exercises you will start to notice shifts in your energy, your thoughts and your feelings. The Lessstressed™ approach to living, is living on your terms, living up to your dreams so that not only can you recover from stress, but you can also start to live a life you love more and more each day.

I know, I did it.

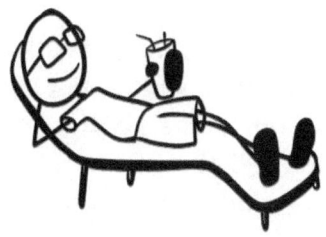

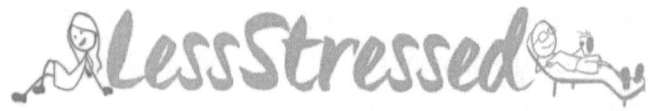

My story of stress

In early 2010, I was off work for 7 weeks with 'stress'. That was what the doctor's notes said – "work related stress". Things weren't good in my marriage either. I call it a breakdown, because it broke down my world and my beliefs about myself.

I'd been on the run for 8 years, since before my children were born. I thought I had 'work /life' balance, but I'd forgotten to put 'me' in the picture. I worked part time which meant that I was always short of cash and always feeling guilty for not 'doing' enough at work. My absence from work was a source of frustration for well-meaning colleagues and I would find myself emailing and working in my 'free' time in order to appease my guilt.

I would feel guilty about being a working mum. My mum didn't work until I was 11, but I went back to work, albeit part time, when both of my sons were 7 months old. I felt sad about leaving them, resentful that I had to, guilt ridden that I was doing them some kind of long term harm. I was the parent who got up with them through the night, when they were ill, during potty training. It was me who organised play dates, swimming lessons and days out.

I also felt like I had to be the chief, the person in charge of all affairs domestic. All I could see was how much I was doing and how much I carried in my head that I had to do - lists and lists of doing, doing, doing. I didn't notice that the fun was going, going, going or that my energy was dull and distant.

I felt torn by my conflicting feelings about the roles I played. I hated house work – I found it boring and endless and thankless and yet I knew that a 'good' wife and mother should be doing a much better job of it than I was. I loved my work and the positive feedback and attention I got and still get from it.

I also wanted to be apple pie 'mom', like the mother on The Waltons, a television programme I loved when I was growing up. She had a handful of children who were all healthy and vital and she would cook huge family dinners whilst listening to her teenager's problems, having just weaned a lamb or harvested apples. I wanted to grow my own vegetables (which end up being over grown by weeds), cook home-made meals (which although edible, were rarely inspirational) and cakes (which at times would have made better kitchen tiles!) and have a house full of children playing and mums chatting (this bit I do well!)

I now see that so much of who I was and what I was doing at that time came from my Ego.

I can see now that I was so tied up with having a nice clean house, being the perfect 'Country Living' housekeeper, Supportive Wife, Nurturing and Endlessly Giving Mother, Professional, and worrying about what other people thought of me that I was lost, exhausted and out of touch with myself.

 When I look back on that time, I remember the thoughts I was running through my head: 'I deserve a promotion', 'why can't they see how good I am', 'look at me do all of this and praise me', 'I'm better than these other people', 'No one can do what I do', 'they would never manage without me'. I was *striving* for attention, *expecting* to be noticed and *trying* so hard to be better and better at everything just so other people would notice and then I would feel good. 'Striving', 'expecting' and 'trying' are so much hard work and without pleasure or joy. They are all linked to the future and to other people.

These thoughts about what I *should* be, and what I wanted other people to see of me were the masks; they cost me greatly though as I never did feel loved enough or good enough. Deep down I felt that people only loved me for the mask and not for the shaky, flaky, insecure, frightened person I felt inside. At work, although I was internally demanding praise and recognition, those demands came from an even more internal place of not feeling good enough, not up to the job. I was so wrapped up in what life and people 'should' be like, that I wasn't paying attention to how life was.

I didn't notice that my moods were getting worse. I was hurried and harried and wouldn't allow myself to stop. Eric Berne says that harried is a 'game', a way of avoiding intimacy:

> 'This game is played by the harried housewife. Her situation requires that she be proficient in ten or twelve different occupations...mistress, mother, nurse, housemaid, etc. These roles are usually conflicting and fatiguing...whose symptoms can succinctly be summarized in the complaint: 'I'm tired' ' (The Games People Play, 1964. p88)

I was also telling myself 'I can't have fun and enjoy myself until all the work and looking after other people is done'. And of course it never was all done, so I never did enjoy myself. In the end the masks and all my striving and expectations just wore me out and as I 'broke down' all the masks fell off and my mind went blank. I could do nothing. Decide nothing. There we no thoughts in my head and I couldn't stop crying. I hid in the toilet so the kids wouldn't see me but they did and brought me their teddies which made me feel like a bad mother and even more guilty so I cried some more.

All of the masks, I can now see, were linked in with pleasing other people, by doing what I thought they thought I *should* do – but I never asked what they wanted from me. I tried to please them as I thought making them happy would make me happy. Keep work happy, my children happy, my husband happy. But I forgot about me.

So, on day three of crying (and painting the hall bright pink!), I realised that it was the first time I had had time to myself in 8 years. The first time I could just cry and scribble in my diary and go for walks and not pick up the phone or check my emails.

- **When was the last time you had time for you?**
- **When did you take the time to do something that you really WANTED to do, rather than something you 'should be doing'.**
- **What are the things you *want* to do just for you?**
- **Could you list them?**

Ignore all the excuses your inner gremlins might make – just keep writing – however outrageous or impossible they seem. Are there any you could start to add into your life now? If not just imagine a time when you can. Could you do one of them for just five minutes a day for a week? How would you benefit it you did some of what you wanted? How would other people benefit from you doing what you wanted?

In my life I've been lucky to have met people who are older than me, who I've respected and looked up to, who have in some way nurtured me, told me their stories and offered for me models for how I might live. They encouraged me on the path from stress to the more loving and peaceful place I find myself in today.

You can make that shift too.

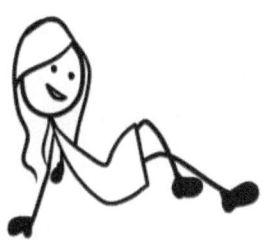

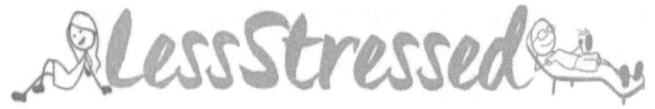

The LessStressed™ approach to living

From Survive and Strive to Revive and Thrive

There are 6 easy steps to a less stressed life.

Step 1 – Understand Stress

You need to understand what stress is and what it does to your body and your mind so that you can spot the signs and symptoms and make changes. It also helps to know it is not just you who gets headaches or a funny tummy or is bad tempered and that there is a biological explanation for why you are feeling so bad.

Once you know how you change when you are stressed then you can look at what your current coping strategies are and decide whether they are helping you or not.

Step 2 – Reduce your stressors

Once you know how stress is affecting you and have considered which stress relieving strategies you can use to help you calm down, you are already to look at the things which are causing you stress; stressors. The Stressless approach to life looks for ways of working with stressors and gathering support so you can do so with ease.

Step 3 – Stop stressing yourself

So much of the stress we feel is as a result of the way that we perceive the situation and when we can change our thoughts, we can change our stress levels. This is really useful when we can't change the stressors; for example, we may not be able to avoid having to commute each day, but we can change how we think about it.

Step 4 – Emotions and stress

You might feel overwhelmed by emotions when you are feeling stressed, or you might feel numb and have no awareness of your emotions at all. This step helps you make friends with your feelings; whatever they are.

Step 5 – You are not your stress

This step teaches you techniques so you can become aware that you are not your stress – what a relief!

Step 6 – Prevent future stress

Stress is often the result of living a life which is out of line with who we are and what we value and so this final step picks you up and turns you around to move increasingly away from stress and towards a life that makes your heart sing.

Ready for a taster of how you can feel less stressed, starting from this moment, right now.

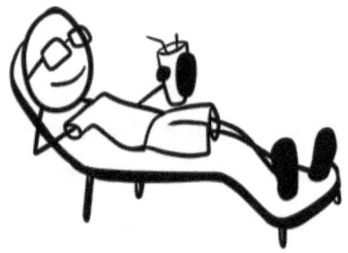

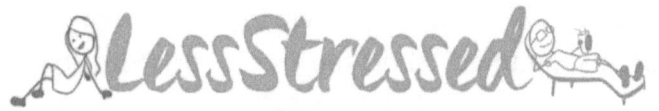

Step 1 – Understand stress

Stress is caused when *perceived* demands outweigh our *perceived* ability to meet them. So if you were to ask me to perform a piano solo in front of you, I would find that stressful as I don't play the piano so the demand would be too high.

However if you asked and accomplished pianist to play for you, they at least in theory, should find it less stressful as they know how to play.

The key words in the first sentence are in italics; 'perceived'. If the accomplished pianist feels that they can't play in front of you, then even though technically they could, they would feel stress as they don't *think* they can.

So some stress is external to us and some is internal.

Some stress is helpful. Eustress is positive stress; the kind of adrenaline buzz which helps you perform well or feel excited.

However dis-stress is when we feel distressed or bad about something. Short term stress or acute stress is an evolutionary response to danger. If a car pulls out in front of you, it is your amygdala that perceives a threat and slams on the breaks thereby saving your life. This is the part of the brain that would have helped our ancestors fight of lions and bears and is part of our fight, flight, freeze or flock response to perceived danger.

When we experience acute stress we produce adrenaline and nor-adrenalin and these and other chemicals in our body make our heart pound, our muscles tense and our breathing quicken all to prepare us to go into battle or run away. After the threat has passed, our parasympathetic nervous system kicks in and helps us calm down.

Long term stress or chronic stress is the killer. It lowers our immunity, slows healing time and is associated with heart disease as the cortisol released hardens our arteries. Long term stress is that job that you hate, the relationship that makes you unhappy, the poverty you live in. This stress does not have the sharp panic of the immediate threat nor does it have the 'phew it's all over' relaxation time; it just goes on and on eroding our wellbeing.

We are usually aware of an acute stress attack such as having someone shout at you, or having your phone stolen. We know what the threat was and we know it has passed.

Chronic stress can be so much part of our daily life that we don't even know we are feeling it; we become habituated to feeling stressed; it becomes the norm. Therefore it is critical to become aware of your signs and symptoms of stress so that you can spot it and do something about it. Whilst we are all different and will experience stress differently, all of the signs and symptoms below have a biological and evolutionary cause.

Stop for a moment and highlight the signs and symptoms you are aware that you have when you are stressed in the grid below. If you think of others that you experience then of course add them in:

Practical Tool – Signs and Symptoms of Stress

Behavioural – your behaviour and actions	Cognitive – Your thinking
Eating, sleeping and drinking too much or not enough	Can't think straight.
	Lots of negative thoughts
Self-harm	Can't make decisions
Failing to do all the things you would usually do	Confused
	Distracted
	Can't focus
Clumsy and accident prone	Forgetful
Engaging in risky activities	
Compulsive behaviours	
Emotional	**At work or studies**
Tearful	Missing deadlines
Angry	Under-performing
Sad	Time off work
Scared	Poor communication
Confused	Conflict at work
Anxious	Low self-esteem
Frustrated	lateness
Irritable	

Physical – your body	Relational – how you react to people
Headache	Blaming and shaming yourself and others
heart pounding	
Tummy ache	Withdrawn
muscles tight	Argumentative
Diarrhoea	Critical
fast, shallow breathing	Promiscuous
Back ache	Distant
clenched teeth	Unkind or uncaring
Hot sweats	Shouting
Dry mouth	
Feel sick	
Tired	
Hyper	

So, now you've spotted some of your signs and symptoms we can start to think about what you are already doing to help you cope with the stress. Most of the time we carry on with life even when we are stressed and we might use strategies that are unhelpful to us. Unhelpful strategies are things and behaviours which might feel great in the short term but leave us feeling bad or sad in the long term. Healthy behaviours are behaviours which support our health and wellbeing in the long term as well as the short term and we feel better for having done them.

Practical Tool – Coping Strategies

Here is a list of common coping strategies; do you recognise that you use any of these? Are there any other coping strategies you use? Can you categorise them?

HELPFUL AND HEALTHY	UNHELPFUL AND UNHEALTHY	HAS NO GREAT AFFECT
Running A hot bath Talking to friends Listening to music Meditation Eating well Solving the problem	Wine Chocolate Bitching and complaining Shopping Work avoidance Over spending	Watching East Enders Ignoring the problem

How can you do fewer of the unhelpful coping strategies and boost the helpful and healthy ways of coping?

Coping is a way of managing stress when it is present, but it isn't a solution, so let's move on to look at the changes you can make to permanently reduce stress in your life.

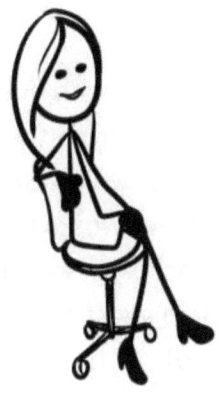

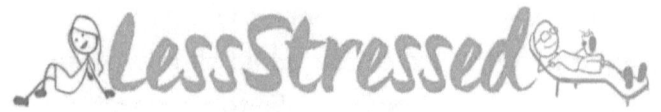

Step 2 – Reduce your stressors

Stressors are the things that are causing us stress, like those illustrated below.

Create your own map like this one with every stressor as a line or spoke coming from the centre of the circle to the edge. Then decide on a scale; it could be 1-10 or 1-100, whatever works for you. Give yourself a number for each stressor; so for example, on this diagram the biggest stressor is 'the boss' coming in with a score of 35/35. The least stressful thing is 'the kids' with a score of 7/35.

Practical Tool – Stressor Map

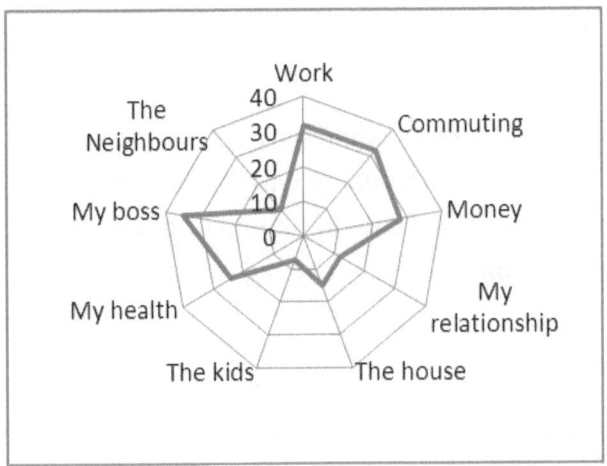

When you look at your own map you will have a clear image of the areas of your life which you see as stressful. For example the map above seems to suggest that work and money are the causes of stress whereas home is OK.

Once you have identified the main sources of your stress, break them down further. So for example; I asked the client above which aspects of work were causing the most stress which is why we then added in 'the boss' as it was this relationship that was the major stressor; there were other areas of work which my client enjoyed.

Once you have identified the aspects of the stressors, think about which aspects you can change, avoid, adapt or delegate. 'Change' means a completely change, for example the client above considered moving jobs.

In the end though he decided to 'adapt' which was to think of ways to communicate with his boss to minimises stress as he couldn't avoid or delegate every interaction. However, he did avoid the commuting nightmare by changing his working hours which considerably lowered his stress.

Practical Tool – Manage those Stressors

Now classify your stressors in the following table:

CHANGE	ADAPT	DELEGATE	AVOID

Sometimes we need help and this might be in the form of getting support from other people or it might simply mean that we need more information or resources. So the client above looked into car sharing and found that no one lived near him but when he talked to HR they were happy for him to go in to work early and leave early so he could miss the rush hour.

Practical Tool – Get Support with your Stressors

What do you need to help you with each?

Stressor	Resources – things I need	Support- people who can help
Eg Commuting	Research car-sharing	HR at work Partner Rail company colleagues

Practical Tool – Take Action Time Line

Once you are clear on what help you need to change you stressors, create a clear time line of actions to take and dates by which you will have taken them.

By Monday	A week on Friday	By the start of next ˌ
Research train times	Talk to HR about changing work ˌ	Start work at 7 and finish at 3

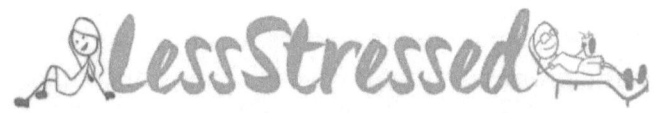

Step 3 – Stop stressing yourself

Sadly, not all stressors can be avoided or at least not straight away. So my client couldn't just change jobs (although he started looking). So some stressors need to be dealt with in another way.

If you remember at the start of this book there was a definition of stress which was that stress is caused by the *perceived* demands and our *perceived* ability to meet them. How we *perceive* a situation can cause us stress.

One way to reduce stress is to reframe a situation i.e. to think about it differently. Let's look at another issue I have supported clients with; the menopause.

Women can't control when the menopause starts or ends. We can influence how we experience it through medication, exercise and diet but we can't stop it happening.

We can, however, change how we think about it. Cognitive psychology works on how we think about the world and how this influences how we live. Its basic premise is that if we can change our thoughts we can change our feelings and our behaviours.

There are of course some situations where we need to change our life. Changing how we think about living with someone who scares us is not as effective as leaving. Changing how we think about a job we hate will not make us as happy as finding work we love.

But when we can't change anything then changing our thinking can turn an inevitable experience from a negative one to a positive one.

I asked my client to talk through all the thoughts she was having about the menopause without censoring and here are some of the common thing she and other women say:

- *I'm getting old*
- *I'm unattractive*
- *No one will find me attractive*
- *Life is over*

These thoughts produce stress and anxiety. Once we have brought these beliefs out into the open, we play a game with them. We start to find evidence to argue against our beliefs for example:

I'm getting old
- But not as old as I will be tomorrow, or the day after, or the year after. In fact I am only old in comparison to yesterday and last year, I am young in comparison to tomorrow and next year.
- There are other people older than me

I'm unattractive
- I'm no more or less attractive than the day before or the year before, I just have a few more lines on my face
- I am as attractive as other people
- My friend told me I looked good the other day

When we start to argue with our thoughts we can see that there are other possible ways of perceiving a situation and this can free up energy and lessen stress by changing perception.

Then we work on building up alternative positive thoughts such as:

- *No more periods*
- *I won't need contraception*
- *I can pay attention to what I need and not worry about anyone else*

Theory - Albert Ellis – ABC

Albert Ellis was a cognitive psychologist and he became interested in the way that our thinking affects our thinking and behaviour.   He invented the ABC model drawing on ideas from philosophy as well as psychology.

Here is a quick overview of his model:

A= **Activating event –** what actually happens

B= our **Beliefs** about what happened which leads to…

C= the **Consequence,** i.e. how we respond to what happened.

For example:

A – I don't get invited out because I'm not in a couple

B – I think everyone hates me and I have no friends

C- So I feel bad about myself and withdraw even more from social contact.

Ellis went on to say that when we are having unhelpful beliefs that harm us, we need to **D= dispute** them by finding counter evidence. So for the example above I might challenge my belief that 'everyone hates me' and find examples of people who like me, I might ask the people who didn't invite me out why they didn't. This would be 'evidence' to dispute the belief.

I could also think of other reasons why I wasn't invited; maybe they didn't think I would be up for it, maybe they felt awkward about me being on my own or maybe they just forgot to invite me. I can't change the **Activating event**, but if I change my **Beliefs** about the situation, then I change the **Consequences**.

So if I change the belief from 'everyone hates me and I have no friends' to 'they just weren't sure if I would want to go and so didn't ask' then the Consequence changes so that I feel better about myself and about them and will be more likely to get in touch with them or talk to them if we bump into each other.

- **Can you think of a situation recently where your Belief has been negative or unhelpful and so has created stress**
- **Can you dispute that belief?**
- **How does it feel when you change the belief for a new one?**

Theory - Negative Automatic Thoughts (NATS)- Aaron Beck

Aaron Beck was another cognitive theorist and therapist and he claimed and proved in his work that depression is linked to how we think. He couldn't prove whether NATs caused the drop in serotonin or whether the drop in serotonin cause the NATs, but we know that there is a link.

A NAT is a negative thought that we often don't even know we are having. NATs can be so ingrained or so frequent that we can be unaware of them, or if we are aware of them, we believe that they are true. Here are some examples of common NATs:

- I'm not good enough
- I can't do it
- I'm stupid/ ugly/fat/ useless
- It's my fault
- It's hopeless
- Life will never change

- **Do you recognise any of those beliefs in yourself?**
- **Do you have any other NATs? (they might not seem like 'beliefs' they might seem 'true'.**

- **Create a list of all your NATs**
- **What NATs are you having about your stressors?**

Practical Tool – NAT catching

When Beck worked with his clients he would give them homework and one of the homeworks was what he called 'thought catching'. Thought catching is when we start to notice what we are thinking more and more.

As you go through the day, keep the list with you and whenever you become aware of what it is you are thinking, make a note.

At the end of the day, have a look at your list.

- **Do you notice any repetition and thought patterns (e.g. are you always thinking about how under-appreciated you are at work or how incompetent people are?)**
- **How many of your thoughts are positive and helpful to you?**
- **Underline or highlight any negative, unkind or unhelpful thoughts.**

Add to your thought catching list every day for a week and then at the end of that time, week ask yourself the questions above for the whole week.

You will start to see patterns. Once you start to see the negative beliefs you are regularly having, you can start to challenge them. In order to challenge our NATs or our Beliefs we need evidence from our own life but also from the outside world and asking other people is one way to get evidence from the outside world.

When we change our thinking, we can change how we behave and how we feel. If I tell myself that I hate my job then I will find things to hate each day and will make myself miserable. If I tell myself that there are bits of my job that I don't like and then look at the things I do like then I will make myself happier without changing a thing. So we can reduce stress by changing how we think about things.

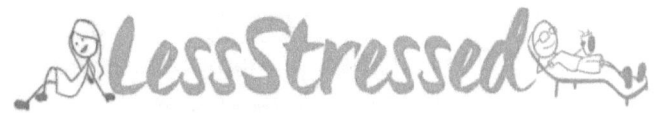

Step 4 – Your Emotions and stress

Sometimes changing our thinking is not enough to change our feelings. As babies, our emotions run unchecked, we cry when we are hungry or tired and we chuckle when something is funny. As we get older and come up against a world of social conditioning, we may adapt our emotions to fit in. Boys learn not to cry or be vulnerable and girls learn not to show anger or pride.

We categorise emotions into 'nice' and 'not nice' or 'good' and 'bad' and develop beliefs that we should feel the good emotions and not the bad. However, all emotions are part of being human and learning to make them our friends can greatly reduce stress.

Practical Tool – Lean In

Often when we are feeling stressed we add to that stress by telling ourselves that we shouldn't be feeling what we are feeling.

So you might be feeling sensitive and overwhelmed if you are stressed and then to add to the emotional pain you judge and blame yourself for feeling sensitive and overwhelmed so then you also feel guilt and shame – perfect! There is another way.

One very simple way to deal with emotions when they come up is simply to lean into them rather than to try and change them or run away from them. Leaning in simply means letting the emotion be, welcoming it and being curious about what it feels like in your body, and what thoughts go with it. Just allow all the sensations of the feeling to be there. If it means crying, cry. If you want to wail, wail. If you want to hit something, get a pillow. If you want to scream and shout get out in the open space and scream and shout (I always find that trees don't mind being screamed at).

If you watch young children, they can be sobbing one minute and giggling the next and they seem to experience each feeling so intensely. That's what leaning in looks like; when we allow each emotion to just be what it is, it passes. We only get stuck in one emotion when we resist it or try to change it. Children don't feel guilty that they feel sad, they just feel sad. They don't feel annoyed at themselves for being tired and crabby, they are just tired and crabby. When we resist an emotion we complicate it and often add another negative emotion (such as guilt and shame) which them makes us feel doubly bad.

Feelings are feelings, they don't have to lead to actions. Just because we feel hatred doesn't mean we should act that out. If you feel jealous, feel jealous. It doesn't mean you have to do anything to the person you are feeling jealous about or to yourself. Nothing has to change just because you are having a feeling. Just notice how it feels, be curious about what it is trying to tell you and let it be. It will pass. All feelings do.

Practical Tool – Feelings as Messengers

Feelings are like messengers, they give us the inside information that our rational brain can't access. Our emotional brain processes information faster than our rational brain. Neither is superior to the other, they both have different roles. When you feel a strong emotion you can bring your rational brain in to investigate your emotional brain.

I went through a stage where I noticed I was having really strong feelings of hatred. I tried to change the feelings by changing my thoughts, by doing affirmations, by distracting myself, but hatred stayed. I didn't like feeling hatred as it didn't fit with my image of myself as being a 'nice' person. When I talked to a male friend about it his blunt reply was 'some people deserve to be hated'. Ah! I'd never before had permission to feel hatred before as somewhere in my past I'd learned that nice people like me don't feel hatred, so it was a shock to feel that yes I did.

So once I'd had permission to feel what I was feeling and stop trying to change how I was feeling then I got curious. My Toltec friend told me to investigate the feeling so I did. I asked myself these questions:

- Where can I feel it in my body? *(Over my heart)*
- What does it feel like? What does it look like? What colour and texture does it have? *(A cold grey stone that was really heavy)*
- What is its purpose? *(To protect my heart, to act as a shield)*

The final question and my answer was such a turn around in how I felt about feeling hatred. In that answer I understood that hatred was actually my friend, it was helping me keep away from someone that had hurt me and could hurt me again. Hatred was acting as my shield to protect my heart – how cool is that?!

Work through those same questions yourself next time you have a strong feeling:

- **Where do I feel it in my body?**
- **What does it look like? Feel like? Colour? Weight? Temperature?**
- **Does it have a sound? Smell? Taste? Texture?**
- **What is its purpose? Ask it with curiosity not judgement.**

Our emotions are on our side if we listen to them and don't distort them by denying or repressing them. Jealousy is often the messenger that helps us clarify what we want, fear reminds us to keep away from danger, sadness lets us know we have lost something that mattered to us.

Anger is a complex emotion and one which I think many of us are brought up not to feel as it's another emotion that can be seen as 'not nice', maybe particularly for girls. When I was doing my PhD research I spoke to children who had been excluded from school, often for swearing at a teacher or fighting. When I asked them questions, it became really clear that boys in particular would get angry when actually they were really feeling sad or scared. They told me that it wasn't 'manly' to show sadness or fear but it was OK to get angry so at an unconscious level they would use anger as a mask for the more vulnerable feelings they were feeling.

I know that some times when I get angry, beneath that I am often feeling scared of not being loved or accepted or sad at being misunderstood or alone.

Anger is what we call a contact emotion; it reaches out to another person to make contact and to be understood. Sadness and fear make us retreat and withdraw into our own world and so their more robust cousin knows that often sadness and fear would be better faced with another person so it goes about its rather blunt and uncouth way to try and get that need for contact met.

Anger is like a big brother who sees that sadness and fear are more vulnerable than him and so goes charging in to fight their corner for them, and in so doing can sometimes make matters worse by pushing people away. So when you are next feeling angry, just ask yourself if there is anything you are sad or scared about as when you make direct contact with those feelings, big brother anger can chill as contact is made.

Anger of course is also a warrior emotion. It guards our boundaries and lets people know when it is time to back off. Whether it is physical boundaries (I get cross when my kids get into my personal stuff), social boundaries (for example when someone lets you down last minute without reason), sexual, intellectual or emotional boundaries; anger will be there to stand up for your rights and assert your territory.

Joy, love, elation, ease, hope, happiness, excitement, pride and passion are all emotions which on the whole we allow ourselves to experience more easily as they are seen as 'positive'. However, sometimes we can even feel guilty about experiencing these emotions.

Again, if we look at young children, they puddle jump between emotions. Splash sadness, another puddle and splash laughter, and another puddle, splash tears, another puddle, splash hitting their brother or sister in rage. They can splash from emotion to emotion minute by minute and each emotions is real and intensely felt. Why? Because they haven't learned not to, and sadly we have.

Our emotions become socialised over time and so we end up being in touch with feelings that we think are acceptable. I did my teacher training with a girl who had been brought up in a religious family who had taught her that this life is suffering and that happiness would be after death. No wonder then that she not only spent a lot of time crying and feeling sad. She hated teaching and would be sick each morning before school. When I asked her what she would love to do, she said that she would love to work in an art gallery...but she couldn't. The main reason she couldn't was that she knew it would make her happy and happiness in her family was not allowed.

We might not be as extreme as that, but I wonder how often you allow yourself to feel joy, elation, bliss, calm, ecstasy, tranquillity?

Practical Tool – Notice, name, depersonalize, let go

When we use this tool, we don't do anything at all, we just notice how we are feeling and let it pass.

Notice and name

Naming the sensations, feelings and thoughts can help us detach from them, to be the observer of them as well as the person experiencing them.

So you might notice:

- **My head hurts**
- **I am feeling despairing**
- **I'm imagining that nothing will ever go right again**
- **I am useless**
- **I am full of self-loathing**
- **I hate the world.**
- **I wish my children would let me have some peace**

How does it feel to actually notice and name what you are experiencing?

We are often so determined to not feel what we are feeling that it can be a relief just to name our experience and acknowledge it.

Depersonalize

Once you've noticed and named what you are feeling, we are then going to remove the 'I' from the experience:

- **There is pain in my head**
- **There is a feeling of despair**

- **There is a thought that nothing will ever go right again**
- **There is a thought that I loathe myself**
- **There is a feeling that I hate the world.**
- **There is a thought that I wish my children would let me have some peace**

This might feel really artificial to start off with, but what the linguistic change does is take 'I' or 'you' further from the experience, without denying the experience. It makes you the observer as well as the person feeling or thinking in the way you are feeling and thinking.

Let it pass through

When we are meditating, we notice how our brain comes up with thought and out body with feelings and sensations and we are invited to just notice them and come back to watching the breath. This is what we are going to do now.

- There is pain in my head **and I know that it will pass**
- There is a feeling of despair **and I know that it will pass**
- There is a thought that nothing will ever go right again **and I know that it will pass**

- There is a thought that I loathe myself **and I know that it will pass**
- There is a feeling that I hate the world **and I know that it will pass.**
- There is a thought that I wish my children would let me have some peace **and I know that it will pass**

Again, this might feel weird to start off with, but as we practice we start to notice that yes of course these thoughts and feeling and experiences pass; everything does.

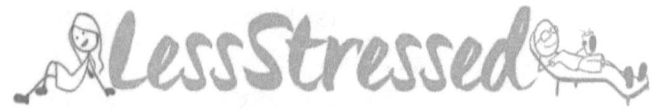

Step 5- You are not your stress

As you go through this book we are going more deeply inward, away from the outside world and into your thoughts and feelings and now we're going to go deeper still and shift stress by noticing that you are not your thought or your feelings or your stress. You are the consciousness noticing your stress, your thoughts and your feelings! You are the person that was noticing your feelings passing through.

This can sound mind-blowing so try out these simple tools and see for yourself.

Practical Tool – Meditation

Meditation, in its very simplest form is the practice of watching ones breath. You don't have to sit or lie in any particular way although it helps to have your lungs able to breathe freely. All you do is tune into your breathing and pay attention to it as it comes and goes.

It sounds so simple, and of course isn't and also it is.

Just find a quiet place and sit comfortably. Shut your eyes and notice your breathing without changing it. Pay attention to the area between your top lip and your nose and feel the air cross it. Feel the breath as it hits the back of your throat and notice it as your chest rises and your stomach expands.

Your mind will want to keep worrying, planning, going back over things, writing lists, and doing what minds do: think, often the same thoughts over and over again. This happens all the time it's just that when we are meditating we notice what we are thinking.

When you notice that your mind has wondered away from watching your breath; then gently bring it back to the breath. You won't stop your thoughts coming and going, but you can let them come and go without you having to get caught up in them.

Watch your breath. When your attention wanders off to a thought, a physical feeling, a noise, a smell, as soon as you have noticed that your attention has wondered, bring it back to the breath.

That's it. That's all you have to do, so easy and yet so tricky. The practice is the point so give up any idea of being 'good at' meditation. The point of meditation is the doing of it.

The more you practice the more you will notice how your thoughts come from nowhere and disappear to nowhere, so do your emotions and your bodily sensations. We are in a permanent state of change and flux.

When we realise this, we begin to see more clearly, that not only do we not have to believe our thoughts or react to our feelings, but that we don't need to because nothing lasts for long. We begin to notice when we are not stressed and when we are not worrying and when we do we can no longer tell ourselves 'I am stressed' because you can see that whilst that might be true for one minute, it might not be true the next.

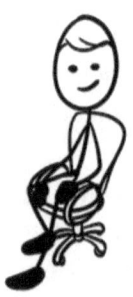

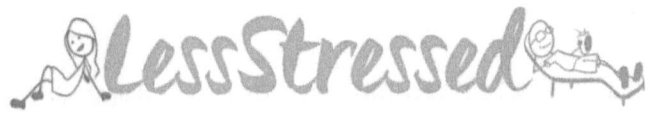

Step 6 – Preventing future stress

Once we realise that we are not our thoughts or our feelings, we can be more playful in the face of things we used to think of as stressful. In fact, we can just side step stress and create a different way of living so that peace and joy are more present in our lives.

Practical Tool - Make it Positive

In the cognitive step above we looked at how we can Dispute thoughts which lead us to feel stressed.

Now let's try an exercise which goes beyond disputing negative beliefs, instead let's flip the beliefs completely.

This game draws on the work of two great women. Nancy Kline is a life coach and in her book; 'Time to Think' she explains how she asks clients to list their assumptions and then to look at the positive opposites of them. Byron Katie plays with the same idea and extends it by asking clients to 'turn it around' not just to find the positive opposite, but to find other ways of saying it.

Let's play.

Take a thought or assumption which is causing you stress. For example:

- My kids should tidy their room
- My partner should give me more hugs

Now let's find the positive opposite assumptions behind each

- My kids do tidy their room
- My partner does give me hugs

Now although these positive opposites might at first sight seem 'untrue', have another look and see if there isn't some truth in them after all. Do your kids sometimes tidy their room or areas of their room? Does your partner sometimes hug you?

Now let's turn those thoughts around further

- My kids shouldn't tidy their room
- I should tidy their room
- I shouldn't tidy their room
- Their room is tidy
- Their room shouldn't be tidy

As you turn your complaint around, just notice what the truth is in the alternatives; maybe their room is tidy but your expectations are too high? Maybe their room shouldn't be tidy because they are kids? Keep looking for truth in the turn arounds.

- My partner should give me more hugs
- My partner shouldn't give me more hugs
- My partner gives me more hugs than I give him
- I should give him more hugs
- We hug the right amount
- I don't like hugs

The key thing here is to make active choices to find the many truths about the same situation. We can get so fixed into one way of seeing things and this can be stressful and yet when we play this game we can see that there are multiple truths operating and one time. So you can want more hugs from your partner AND realise that he hugs you more than you hug him AND realise that you could hugs him more all at the same time.

Then we can switch our focus again. Instead of finding stressors and changing them and our beliefs, we can just train our brain to notice different things. We now know that our brain can constantly be rewired and we can consciously train our brain to look for the positive and the pleasurable in our life more and more.

Practical Tool - What Went Well diary

This is a tool I learned from a workshop run by with the Centre for Applied Positive Psychology at Warwick University. It works in the same way as the affirmations as it encourages us to rewire our brain by choosing to focus on the positive.

All you have to do is write down all and as many of the following; try answering the questions for today so far:

- **What went well?**
- **What you did well?**
- **What you enjoyed?**
- **What you appreciated?**
- **What brought you happiness and pleasure?**
- **What are all the good things that you have in your life?**

Some days it can be hard to think about anything that felt like it was going well. After a bereavement or a redundancy we feel so overwhelmed with the sadness or fear that it is hard to notice anything positive. And yet even on these days there is still air to breathe, the earth to stand on, and our lives to live. On these days you have to look hard, look at the detail, look at the things you take for granted. What did you do well? Did you get the kids up on time, did you make breakfast? Did you get to work? Did you walk the dog? Have a shower? Make something to eat? Then notice and give yourself credit for those things.

What did you appreciate? Did you notice your children's smiles, did you pay attention to the fact that a friend called or a colleague asked how you were? Did you appreciate having a hot meal at work, or that the train ran on time. These are the thing that day in and day out happen without us noticing until they go wrong. Let's notice and appreciate them when they go well.

What are all the good things you have in your life? A home? Hot water? Food? Health? Friends? A warm bed? Pets? Kids? Again, in our culture we have so much to be grateful for and we take so much for granted so pay attention to the all that you have.

The more you do this, the more you will notice things that you appreciate and things that you do well and the more you notice those things the better you will feel. This isn't to say that irritations won't occur or sadness won't appear; there is enough space for all your feelings and still to be appreciative.

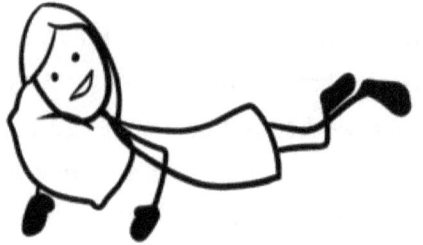

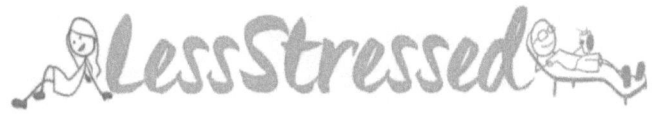

Conclusion

Stress makes us unhappy, it makes us ill and it shortens our life expectancy. Life can be challenging and there will always be things which we can change or adapt or stop doing which will make our life more easeful. When we can't change our external world, we can change our internal world; we can notice that we are more than our stress and more than our fears. Noticing that we are stressed can be the first step to turning our thoughts, feelings and lifestyle into a life which is more alive; a life in which we can thrive rather than just survive and strive. Practice these tools and approaches and see a your life flourish.

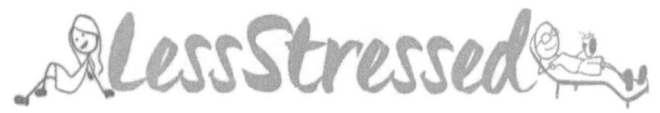

Next steps

If this eBook has been helpful then pop over to www.lessstressed.co.uk and check out the coaching, training and resources to help you on your way to lessstressed™ living.

If you are stressed because of relationship difficulties or domestic abuse you will find resources and support at www.lovebeingme.co.uk

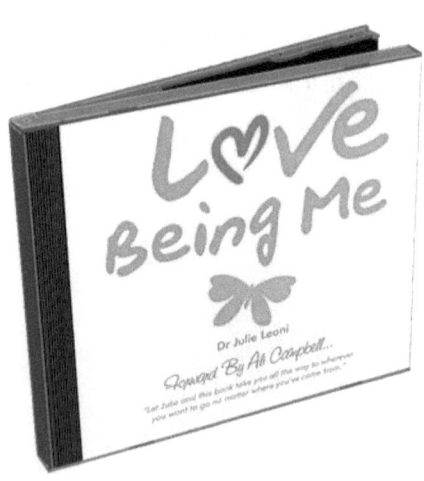

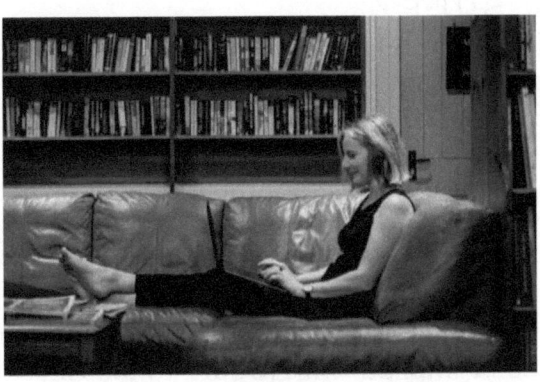

Julie Leoni is the creator of the LessStressed™
Approach to Living. She is also an author, life
coach and psychology teacher with years of
experience of training and facilitating groups.
She has worked with organisations to develop
Emotional Intelligence and has experience and
training in bereavement, domestic abuse,
mindfulness and meditation as well as a number
of therapeutic approaches. She has 2 sons who
she loves loads and who sometimes drive her
crazy.
Web: **www.lovebeingme.co.uk**
Web: www.lessstressed.co.uk
Email::julie@lovebeingme.co.uk

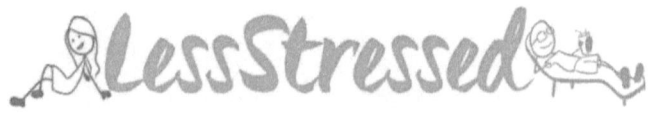

individual's success will be determined by his or her desire, dedication, motivation, effort, previous life experience and individual personality. There are no guarantees that you will achieve the results described herein nor is there a time frame within which any personal change might happen.

The intent of the author is only to offer information of a general nature to help you in your quest for emotional, intellectual and spiritual well-being. In the event you use any of the information in this book for yourself, the author assumes no responsibility for your actions. Also, you should use this information as you see fit, and at your own risk. Your particular situation may not be exactly suited to the examples illustrated here; in fact, it's likely that they won't be the same, and you should adjust your use of the information and recommendations accordingly.

(1) Ownership of copyright
The copyright in this eBook and the material on this website (including without limitation the text, computer code, artwork, photographs, images, music, audio material, video material and audio-visual material on this website) is owned by Julie Leoni, Love Being Me and our licensors.

(2) Copyright licence
We grant to you a worldwide non-exclusive royalty-free revocable licence to:

(a) View this eBook and website and the material in the eBook and on this website on a computer or mobile device via a web browser;
(b) Copy and store this eBook and website and the material in this eBook and on this website in your web browser cache memory; and
(c) Print pages from this eBook and website for your own [personal and non-commercial] use.
We do not grant you any other rights in relation to this eBook and website or the material in this eBook and on this website. In other words, all other rights are reserved.
For the avoidance of doubt, you must not adapt, edit, change, transform, publish, republish, distribute, redistribute, broadcast, rebroadcast or show or play in public this eBook or website or the material in this eBook and on this website (in any form or media) without our prior written permission.

(3) Data mining
The automated and/or systematic collection of data from this eBook and website is prohibited.

(4) Permissions
You may request permission to use the copyright materials in this eBook or website by writing to Julie@lovebeingme.co.uk

(5) Enforcement of copyright
We take the protection of our copyright very seriously. If we discover that you have used our copyright materials in contravention of the licence above, we may bring legal proceedings

against you seeking monetary damages and an injunction to stop you using those materials. You could also be ordered to pay legal costs.

If you become aware of any use of our copyright materials that contravenes or may contravene the licence above, please report this by email to

(6) Infringing material
If you become aware of any material on our website that you believe infringes your or any other person's copyright, please report this by email to Julie@lovebeingme.co.uk
The right of Julie Leoni to be identified as the author of this work has been asserted in accordance with the Copyright, Designs and Patents Act 1988

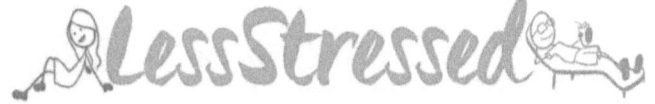